I Know About Germs!

Story by Tedi McVea, LCSW

Illustrated by Noel de la Mora

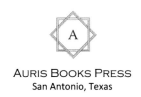

AURIS BOOKS PRESS
San Antonio, Texas

I know all
about germs.....

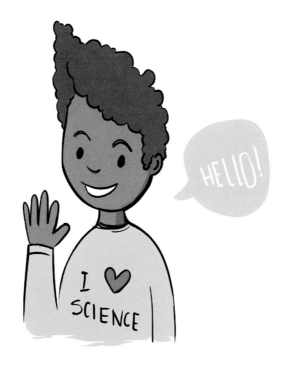

That is because I am
smart and I love science.

Some germs are tiny bad guys that can live on things.

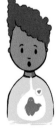

Lots of germs even live in your body!

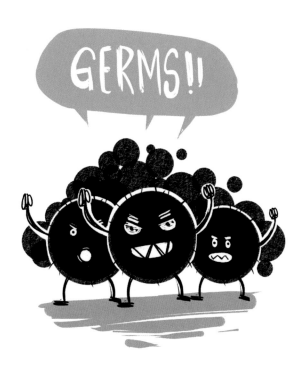

Don't worry!

we have an army of good guys inside of us, too.

They help us fight the bad guys.

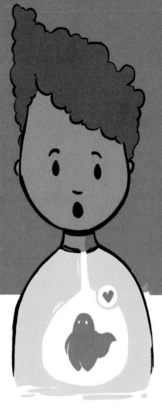

They are just like

SUPERHEROES!

I imagine my superheroes
wear green and pink.

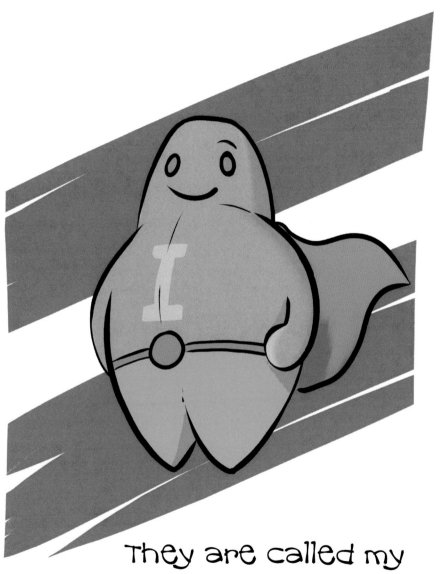

They are called my
Immune system!

Some bad guys
are easy to fight.

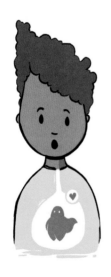

Some are a little harder...

and some are very tricky.

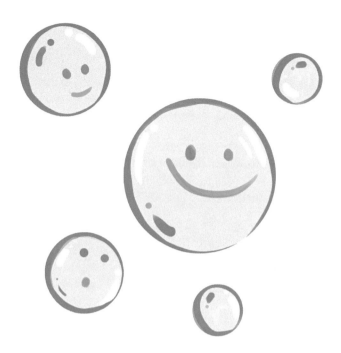

For tricky germs, we have to get just as tricky to fight them back.

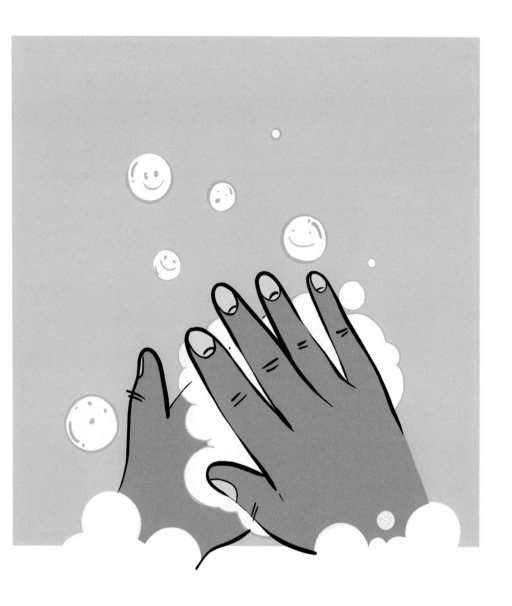

Some really good tricks are to
wash your hands and cover
your mouth when you cough
or sneeze.

These tricks help the superheroes in our body outnumber the bad guys.

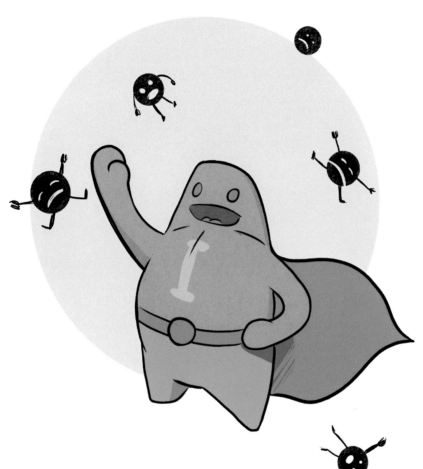

when this happens,
the bad guys can't spread.

Cool, right?

I told you, I know all about science.

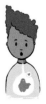

Sometimes, we have to fight very tricky germs that are novel.

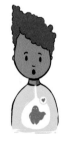

Novel means "new".

Our immune system isn't quite sure how to fight these new germs.

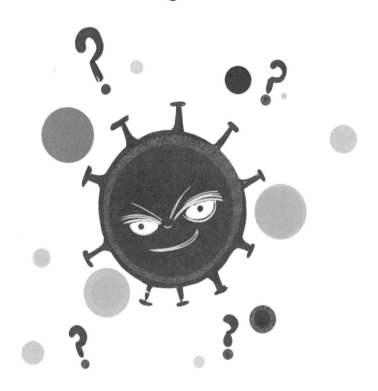

These new germs might know too many tricks.

They know how to spread ... and how to really hurt people.

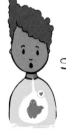

Some germs are really fast!

They can be real
bad guys!

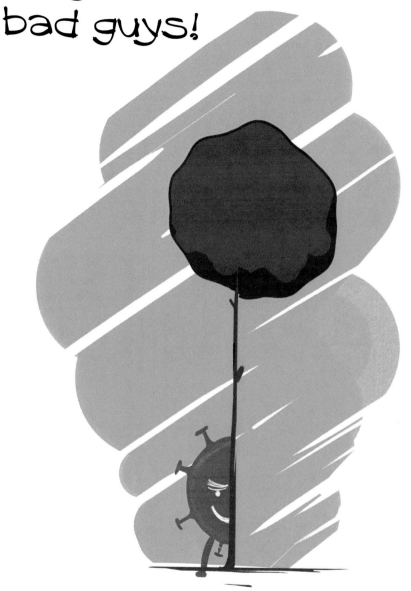

Maybe even the worst!

With new viruses, we have to
be super careful to keep
everyone safe and healthy.

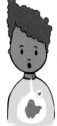

Some germs can spread from person
to person all over the world.

We can't let a
new virus
Try any of its
 favorite tricks.

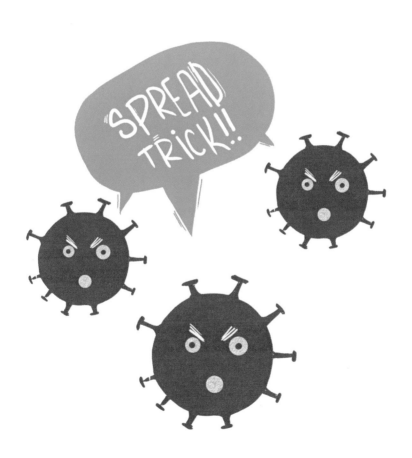

you can help!

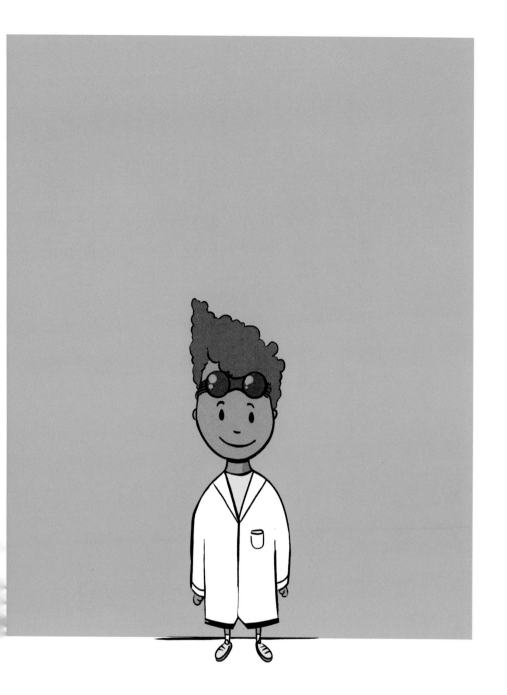

I can teach you all about science.

First, do your best to stay home.

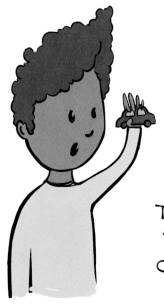

This may even mean not going to school, going shopping, or even going visiting.

That way, the virus can't catch you.

And you can be more careful by not touching your face.

 Don't forget to wash your hands!

Also, talk to your friends and family on the phone.

'HELLO!?'

School might seem different, but you can study on a computer or read books.

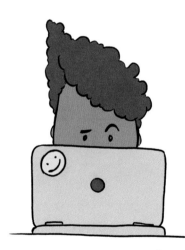

It will not feel the same, but it will still be fun...

...and it will not be forever.

That's called "social distancing."

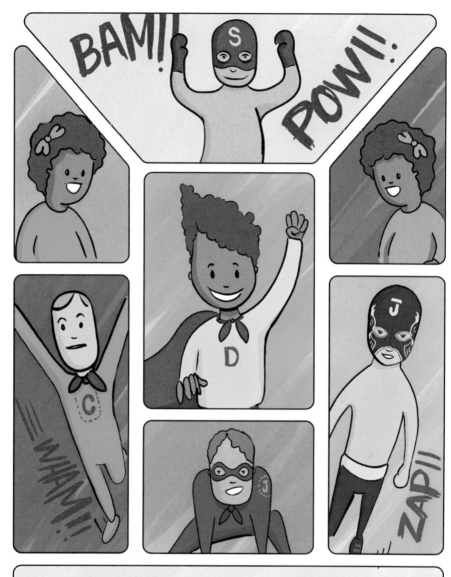

Together, we can help our good guys win this fight! Now, I think you know all about germs, too!

Don't forget to tell your grown-ups!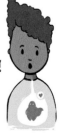

About the Author:
Mother, photographer and clinical social worker, Tedi McVea is the founder of **Mom-ease Bear** (https://www.mom-easebear.com), a platform for mothers nationally to inform and share on their experiences in parenthood.

About the Illustrator:
Born and raised in Guadalajara, Mexico, Noel de la Mora is an accomplished illustrator and 3-D artist. He is art director and founder of several art studies and enjoys traveling in search of new art.

MCVEA, TEDI
DE LA MORA, NOEL

I KNOW ABOUT GERMS

Partial proceeds from sales of this book go to support the Auris Project, Inc., a 501c3 non-profit organization whose mission is to help communities access key rights and development information. For more information, visit us at https://www.aurisproject.org.

For quantity sales or permission requests, please write to Auris Books Press at:

publishing@aurisproject.org

AURIS BOOKS PRESS
San Antonio, Texas

Made in the USA
Middletown, DE
02 September 2021

47494635R00018